Hand Inju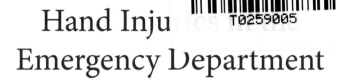ies in the Emergency Department

This new pocketbook introduces students, junior doctors, and clinicians to the vital skills of diagnostic strategy and clinical reasoning for hand injuries. 30% of the patients in an emergency department present with hand injuries or acute non-traumatic problems of the hand. These are rarely life-threatening but can lead to high morbidity and disability due to inadequate diagnosis and treatment resulting in malpractice claims. This book is an easy-to-use ready reckoner for physicians working in ER departments and residents or fellows exposed to hand surgery. It addresses the needs of its core readers and encourages them to refine their powers of observation during physical examination.

Key Features:

- Presents the content in a comprehensive and logical manner with an appropriate level of illustrations.
- Serves as a ready reference of clinical examination in an easy-to-use pocket-book format for residents and physicians who encounter hand injuries.
- Covers crucial knowledge in the field of hand trauma.

Hand Injuries in the Emergency Department

Peter Houpt

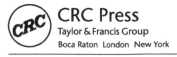

CRC Press

Taylor & Francis Group

Boca Raton London New York

CRC Press is an imprint of the
Taylor & Francis Group, an **informa** business

First edition published 2023
by CRC Press
6000 Broken Sound Parkway NW, Suite 300, Boca Raton,
FL 33487-2742

and by CRC Press
4 Park Square, Milton Park, Abingdon, Oxon, OX14 4RN

CRC Press is an imprint of Taylor & Francis Group, LLC

ISBN: 978-1-032-32243-8 (hbk)
ISBN: 978-1-032-32242-1 (pbk)
ISBN: 978-1-003-31354-0 (ebk)

DOI: 10.1201/9781003313540

Typeset in Minion
by SPi Technologies India Pvt Ltd (Straive)

Contents

Preface

Patients with hand injuries or acute non-traumatic problems of the hand are usually referred to the emergency department.

These are rarely life-threatening conditions, but injury can lead to high morbidity and disability. Inadequate diagnosis and treatment can lead to malpractice claims.

The vast majority of patients are primarily seen by sometimes inexperienced, young physicians. This booklet is mainly written for them, but I hope other professionals who encounter hand injuries will also find this booklet useful. Years ago, the content was reviewed by a number of experienced hand surgeons until consensus was reached.

Thanks to Laura Jansen, a valued plastic colleague, for helping to translate this booklet. Thanks go also to Maartje Kunen for the medical visuals in the book.

PETER HOUPT
Zwolle, The Netherlands

A Note on the Author

Dr Peter Houpt PhD is a plastic surgeon in the Netherlands. His career in the last 35 years has focused on hand surgery. He was a long-time board member of the Dutch society for surgery of the hand and also occupied a seat on the hand trauma committee of the FESSH. Most of his lectures and publications were devoted to hand surgery, and many students were trained in the domain of hand surgery.

Together with his colleagues, Dr Houpt helped to develop the largest hand center in the Netherlands at the Isala Clinics in Zwolle. It received formal recognition as a hand trauma center from the FESSH council.

During many visits to developing countries, one of Dr Houpt's goals was to treat congenital malformations of the hand. He welcomes the day when hand surgery in itself will be an official speciality in the Netherlands.

Abbreviations

AdP	m. adductor pollicis
ADM	m. adductor digiti minimi
AP	antero-posterior
APB	m. abductor pollicis brevis
APL	m. abductor pollicis longus
ATLS	Advanced Trauma Life Support
CMC	carpo-metacarpal
CPK	Creatine phosphokinase
CRPS I	complex regional pain syndrome type I
CT	computed tomography
CTS	carpal tunnel syndrome
DIP	distal interphalangeal
DMSO	Dimethylsulfoxide
DRU	distal radio-ulnar
ECG	electrocardiogram
ECRB	m. extensor carpi radialis brevis
ECRL	m. extensor carpi radialis longus
ECU	m. extensor carpi ulnaris
EDC	m. extensor digitorum communis
EDM	m. extensor digiti minimi
EIP	m. extensor indicis proprius
EPB	m. extensor pollicis brevis
EPL	m. extensor pollicis longus
FCR	m. flexor carpi radialis
FCU	m. flexor carpi ulnaris
FDM	m. flexor digiti minimi
FDP	m. flexor digitorum profundus
FDS	m. flexor digitorum superficialis
FESSH	Federation of European Societies for Surgery of the Hand
FOOSH	fall on the outstretched hand
FPB	m. flexor pollicis brevis

FPL	m. flexor pollicis longus
HF	hydrogen fluoride
IP	interphalangeal
LDH	Lactate dehydrogenase
LT	lunotriquetral
m	muscle
MCP	metacarpo-phalangeal
MRI	magnetic resonance imaging
ODM	opponens digiti minimi muscle
OP	m. opponens pollicis
PA	pathological
PIP	proximal interphalangeal
PL	m. palmaris longus
PSR	processus styloideus radii
PSU	processus styloideus ulnae
ROM	range of motion
SL	scapholunate
TBSA	total body surface area
TFCC	triangular fibrocartilage complex
UCL	ulnar collateral ligament

Introduction

Hand surgery is specialist work. It requires knowledge of the complex static and functional anatomy of the hand. Recognize your potential limitations in the field of hand surgery. Realize that many injuries of the hand, if it concerned yourself, can make your work as a physician impossible. No patient will blame you if you refer him for further assessment. In this book the term 'hand surgeon' is used. Hand surgery in Europe is a recognized specialism in seven countries. It refers to a surgeon with a proven experience and interest in all aspects of hand surgery; and to one who works within an infrastructure that can provide optimal aftercare. The knowledge level may be demonstrated by passing a European examination in hand surgery. Through inspection and good physical examination, it is possible to determine which structure is damaged. Additionally, an X-ray can be taken on indication. Arterial bleeding can always be stopped by a pressure bandage and elevation. Do not use tourniquets and do not place clamps 'blindly'. If, after inspection, there is an indication for treatment to be continued in the operation theatre, further anesthesia and exploration of the wound in the Emergency Department are contraindicated. In the case of serious injuries, however, it may be beneficial to provide a regional (brachial plexus block) anesthesia in anticipation of surgery. Remember: don't throw anything away!

Remnants can sometimes be used as spare parts. If the injury is limited and the treatment fits within the competence of the Emergency Department physician, the finger or hand can be anaesthetized. Disinfect and cover, but leave a large field to operate. After anesthesia, the wound must first be thoroughly rinsed with saline. Carry out a thorough but sparing debridement. Extend (draw!) incisions to get a good overview. Work according to standard Bruner incisions as much as possible (Figure 1.1). Never make longitudinal incisions over the volar side of the fingers.

More than elsewhere in the body, hand surgery requires a non-traumatic technique. Lift the skin with hooks and not with forceps. In case of tissue loss, especially combined with an open joint or exposed tendons, bone or nerves, a transposition or transplantation of skin is indicated. Secondary healing may be intended in small fingertip lesions, but otherwise often leads to contractures and loss of function. After treatment, arm elevation is required for at least a week.

DOI: 10.1201/9781003313540-1

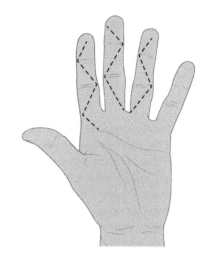

Figure 1.1 Incisions on the volar side of the fingers according to Bruner.

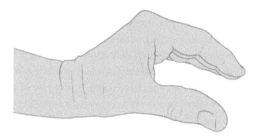

Figure 1.2 'Intrinsic plus' position or 'position of protection'.

Immobilization is a necessary intervention after tendon or ligament injury, or in unstable fractures. If immobilization is decided upon, the 'intrinsic plus' position is preferred (Figure 1.2). The MCP joints are flexed 90° and the IP joints fully extended. This position is also called 'position of protection' and has nothing to do with the functional position. The functional position, as in a ball dressing, is obsolete. Due to the curved position of the IP joints there is a risk of contractures by shortening of the collateral ligaments.

Bunnell's thesis is still accurate to this date:

> As the problem in hand surgery is composite, the surgeon must also be. It is impractical for three specialists (bone, nerve, soft-tissue) to work together or in series. There is no shortcut. The surgeon must face the situation and equip himself to handle any and all of the tissues in a limb.
> (Bunnell 1944)

Anatomy

GENERAL

At the level of the hand and wrist one speaks of the volar (or palmar) side and the dorsal side. The terms ulnar and radial (thumb side) are more straight-forward than medial and lateral. The same applies to the names thumb, index finger, middle finger, ring finger and little finger instead of digitus I to V.

I. Skin

The skin on the palmar side is thicker and more fixed to the sublayer than the elastic, mobile skin of the dorsum of the hand. There is a firm extra layer beneath the palmar skin; the fan-shaped fascia palmaris.

The folds present in the palm of the hand give an indication of the location of the joints.

II. Soft tissues

MUSCLES AND TENDONS

EXTRINSIC MUSCULATURE

FLEXOR TENDONS (FIGURES 2.1–2.3)

Clearly visible on the volar side of the wrist are the tendons of the m. flexor carpi radialis, the m. palmaris longus (which is not present in approximately 20% of the population) and the m.flexor carpi ulnaris (Figure 2.1).

Each finger contains two flexor tendons. These are the m. flexor digitorum superficialis, which attaches to the base of the middle phalanx and is the flexor of the PIP joint, and the flexor digitorum profundus, attached to the base of the distal phalanx and responsible for flexion of the DIP joint. The flexors run in sheaths that are reinforced by thicker areas, also known as pulleys, of which the A2 and A4-pulleys mechanically are the most important for an optimal bending function of the finger (Figure 2.2).

DOI: 10.1201/9781003313540-2

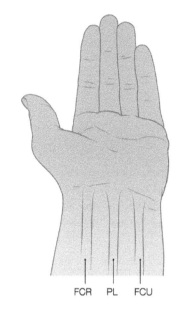

Figure 2.1 Flexor tendons on the volar side of the wrist.

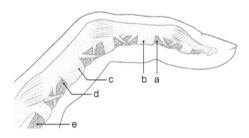

Figure 2.2 The flexor tendons in the finger. a: deep flexor tendon (FDP), b: A4 pulley, c: A2 pulley, d: chiasma of the superficial flexor tendon, e: superficial flexor tendon (FDS).

The thumb contains only one long flexor tendon; the m. flexor pollicis longus. This tendon attaches to the base of the distal phalanx and therefore bends the IP joint.

Volarly, the hand is divided into five zones. These are determined by the relation of the flexor tendons to each other and to the surrounding tissue. For example, zone II is the area where the two flexor tendons are both present

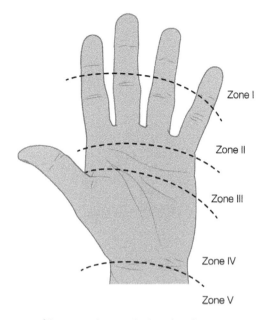

Figure 2.3 Zones of flexor tendons in the hand and wrist.

Zone I

Zone II

Zone III

Zone IV

Zone V

in the tendon sheath of the finger (Figure 2.3). These zones are often used to describe the level of a tendon injury.

EXTENSOR TENDONS (FIGURE 2.4)

At wrist level, the extensor tendons lie beneath the extensor retinaculum and can be divided into six compartments:

First compartment:	m. abductor pollicis longus	(APL)
	m. extensor pollicis brevis	(EPB)
Second compartment:	m. extensor carpi radialis longus	(ECRL)
	m. extensor carpi radialis brevis	(ECRB)
Third compartment:	m. extensor pollicis longus	(EPL)
Fourth compartment:	m. extensor indicis proprius	(EIP)
	m. extensor digitorum communis	(EDC)
Fifth compartment:	m. extensor digiti minimi	(EDM)
Sixth compartment:	m. extensor carpi ulnaris	(ECU)

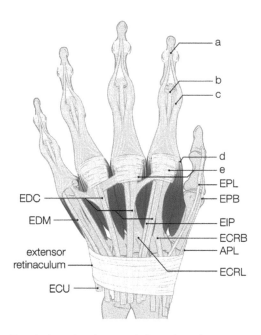

Figure 2.4 a: Terminal tendon, b: central slip, c: lateral component, d: slip from mm. lumbricales and mm. interossei, e: sagittal bands.

The extensors of the thumb form the borders of the anatomical snuff box. The m. extensor pollicis longus lies on the dorsal side of the thumb, inserts onto the distal phalanx and extends the IP joint. The m. abductor pollicis longus and m. extensor pollicis brevis are positioned on the radial side of the anatomical snuff box and provide abduction and extension of the first metacarpal, respectively. Positioned just ulnar to the anatomical snuff box are the two radial extensors of the wrist, the m. extensor carpi radialis longus and brevis, which insert at the base of the second and third metacarpal, respectively. The m. extensor carpi ulnaris is the most ulnar positioned tendon at the level of the wrist. It inserts onto the base of the fifth os metacarpal. The mm. extensor digitorum communis extend the fingers. The index finger has an additional extensor which is located on the ulnar side of the EDC; the m. extensor indicis proprius.

The little finger too consists of a second extensor; the m. extensor digiti minimi/quinti. At the dorsal level of the MCP joints, the extensor tendons are centralized by the sagittal bands. Just distal to this, the extensor aponeurosis divides in a central slip and two lateral slips. The central slip attaches to the base of the middle phalanx and therefore provides extension of the PIP joint. The two lateral slips continue to the base of the distal phalanx where they join and form the terminal tendon. These provide extension of the DIP joint, but proximally also assist in extension of the PIP joint. At the level of the proximal phalanx, the tendons from mm. lumbricales and mm. interossei (the lateral bands) fuse with the two lateral slips.

INTRINSIC MUSCULATURE

Intrinsic muscles are those whose origin and insertion are located within the hand. Located in the thenar eminence are three muscles that together provide opposition (m. opponens pollicis), abduction (m. abductor pollicis brevis) and flexion of the first MCP joint (m. flexor pollicis brevis). The muscles of the hypothenar consist of the m. opponens digiti minimi, m. abductor digiti minimi and the flexor digiti minimi. The thumb is adducted towards the palm by the adductor pollicis, palpated best on the dorsal side of the hand. Located between the metacarpal bones are the mm. interossei. The palmar interossei, three in total, adduct the fingers in the direction of the middle finger. The dorsal interossei, four in total, abduct the fingers away from the middle finger (Figure 2.5). Last but not least the hand contains the mm. lumbricales, which originate from the FDP tendons and insert onto the extensor aponeurosis at the proximal phalangeal level. These lumbrical muscles tighten the extensors such that the fingers can remain extended during the flexion of the MCP joints.

BLOOD VESSELS

The blood supply of the hand is provided by the radial and ulnar arteries, which, in the hand palm, converge to form the superficial and deep vascular arch. The radial artery and ulnar artery in the wrist are positioned on the radial side of the FCR and FCU, respectively. Each finger consists of two digital arteries which lie laterally to the flexor tendons and dorsal to the digital nerve. In the thumb, the digital arteries are more median (thus central) than expected. The thumb has a separate vascularization for the dorsum. Venous drainage takes place through a network of veins that are mainly located on the dorsal side of the hand which proximally drain into the cephalic and basilic vein of the forearm.

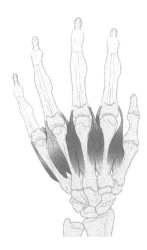

Figure 2.5 The four dorsal mm. interossei.

NERVES

The nerves of the hand are the median nerve, the ulnar nerve and the radial nerve (Figures 2.6 and 2.7).

The **median nerve** runs between the two bellies of the pronator teres muscle in the forearm. It continues between the flexor digitorum superficialis and profundus muscles to the carpal tunnel. During this course it branches off the anterior interosseous nerve to the m. flexor pollicis longus, the m. flexor digitorum profundus of the index finger and m. pronator quadratus. The median nerve itself innervates the m. flexor carpi radialis, the m. pronator teres, the four mm. flexor digitorum superficialis, the m. palmaris longus and the m. flexor digitorum profundus to the middle finger. At the level of the wrist, the median nerve is located on the ulnar side of the FCR and is covered by the palmaris longus tendon. Distally, the median nerve passes through the carpal tunnel underneath the transverse carpal ligament. The motor branch branches off to the thenar and innervates the m. opponens pollicis, the m. abductor brevis and half of the m. flexor pollicis brevis. Finally the median nerve branches off as a sensory nerve to the thumb, index, middle and radial half of the ring finger.

Additionally, it innervates the first and sometimes second m. lumbricalis.

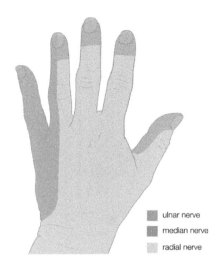

Figure 2.6 Sensory innervation of the dorsal side of the hand.

The **radial nerve** enters the forearm between the two bellies of the m. supinator. It innervates the m. brachioradialis and the m. extensor carpi radialis longus before splitting into the posterior interosseous nerve (a motor nerve) and the superficial radial nerve (a sensory nerve). The posterior interosseous nerve innervates the extensors of the wrist, fingers and thumb. The superficial radial nerve provides sensation to the dorso-radial side of the hand.

The **ulnar nerve** enters the forearm between the two bellies of the m. flexor carpi ulnaris. It innervates the m. flexor carpi ulnaris and the mm. flexor digitorum profundus of the ring finger and the little finger. The ulnar nerve is located on the radial side of the FCU in the wrist and passes through Guyon canal. Distal to this, the nerve splits into motor branches to the mm. interossei, two to three ulnar mm. lumbricales, muscles of the hypothenar, the m. adductor pollicis and half of the m. flexor pollicis brevis. The sensory branches provide the little finger and the ulnar side of the ring finger. Three to four centimeters proximal to the distal wrist crease the ulnar nerve branches off a sensory branch to the ulnar part of the dorsal side of the hand.

As mentioned earlier, the thumb and fingers each have two digital nerves that lie volar to the digital arteries and, depending on the sensory area, originate from the median or ulnar nerve.

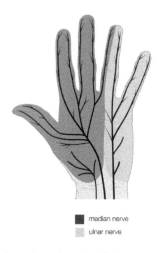

median nerve
ulnar nerve

Figure 2.7 Nerve supply to the volar side of the hand.

BONES OF THE HAND AND WRIST

In the forearm, the radius rotates around the ulna in the distal radio-ulnar joint (DRU joint). The carpal bones of the hand are connected through intrinsic ligaments. The external capsule of the wrist joint is located around the carpalia. Within the carpus, the proximal and distal rows of carpal bones can be distinguished. The os pisiforme is not part of the wrist joint, but acts as a fulcrum for the FCU tendon. In contrast to the fourth and fifth carpometacarpal (CMC) joints, the mobility of the second and third CMC joints is limited. The MCP and IP joints are stabilized by the volar plate and collateral ligaments. The sesamoid bones are located just volar to the MCP joint of the thumb. They sometimes can be located near other joints. The epiphyseal plate is always based proximally in the phalanges of the fingers and distally in the metacarpals, except the metacarpal of the thumb (Figure 2.8).

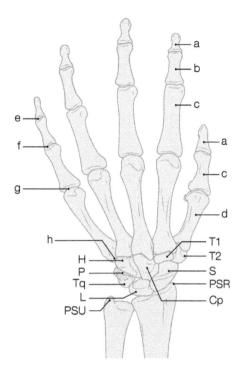

So Long To Pinky Here Comes The Thumb

Figure 2.8 a: distal phalanx, b: middle phalanx, c: proximal phalanx, d: os metacarpal, e: DIP joint, f: PIP joint, g: MCP joint, h: CMC joint, H: os hamatum, Cp. os capitatum, L: os lunatum, S: os scaphoideum, Tq. os triquetrum, P: os pisiforme, T1: os trapezoideum, T2: os trapezium, PSU: processus styloideus ulnae, PSR: processus styloideus radii.

3

Patient history and physical examination

PATIENT HISTORY

Patient

- Age, gender, hand dominance, profession and hobbies.
- Previous illness, injuries or operations of the affected hand.
- Current medication, allergies, tetanus status, intoxications.

Mechanism

- Time, position of the hand at time of accident.
- Method of injury: machine, thickness of saw blade, was the object contaminated?
- Was there any entrapment?
- Was there heat, fire or chemicals involved?

Symptoms

- Pain, numbness, loss of strength, restricted movement

EXAMINATION

To anesthetize the hand before a full examination is carried out (and other than in the context of an operative treatment), is an error. If the hand injury is part of multiple injuries, it is necessary to act in accordance with the principles of the ATLS. The following aspects must be assessed separately:

INSPECTION

Location of the injury: hand, wrist, forearm, elbow, upper arm, shoulder (plexus). Observe the position of the hand and fingers at rest (Figure 3.1) and

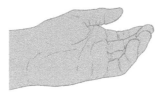

Figure 3.1 Normal hand cascade.

with passive flexion and extension of the wrist (the 'tenodesis effect'). These observations can already hint towards the continuity of the extrinsic flexor and extensor tendons.

Colour: pale, cyanotic, congested or hyperemic
Turgor of the soft tissue
Swelling: edema, hematoma, loss of wrinkling
Presence of foreign bodies
Moist: sweating
Wounds, open joints
Deformities: luxation, fracture

Palpation

Temperature, pain, moisture (a smooth skin can indicate loss of sweat secretion and thus a denervation)
Crepitations, fluctuations, shortening.
Integrity of joint capsule and ligaments: laxity

Physical examination

Always compare with the contralateral unaffected hand or arm. For a general impression of the range of motion of the fingers: ask the patient to make a fist and stretch the fingers, then spread and close. However bear in mind it is still possible to make a clenched fist with all superficial flexor tendons discontinuous. During the physical examination, try to test against resistance. Although subjective, pain can be an indication for a partial tendon injury in which the function may be intact.

EXTRINSIC FLEXORS

FPL: flexion in IP joint, 'bend the top of the thumb'.

FDP: flexion of the distal phalanx, 'bend the top of the finger'. In this investigation the PIP joint is stabilized in extension by the examiner (Figure 3.2).

FDS: flexion of the PIP joint, 'bend your finger in the middle joint'. The remaining fingers are extended by the examiner to disable the FDP function. The middle, ring and little finger have, after all, a common FDP muscle belly (Figure 3.3). For the function test of the FDS of the index finger the patient is asked to make the OK sign.

FCU and FCR: flexion of the wrist, 'bend your wrist'. The tendons must be palpated to identify contraction of a particular wrist flexor, as it is possible to bend the wrist by flexing the fingers.

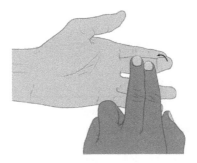

Figure 3.2 Examination of the FDP.

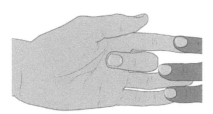

Figure 3.3 Examination of the FDS.

EXTRINSIC EXTENSORS

APL and EPB: hand flat on the table with palm down, ask the patient to move the thumb sideways (abduction). Palpate the tendons at the level of the anatomical snuff box. ECRL and ECRB: ask the patient to make a fist and extend the wrist. Palpate the tendons at the wrist.

EPL: hand flat on the table with palm down, ask the patient to lift the thumb up and out towards the ceiling. Look at the course of the EPL which crosses the second compartment.

EDC and EIP: Ask the patient to extend their fingers in the MCP joints. The EIP can be tested separately by making a fist and only extend the index finger in the MCP joint. It is good to bear in mind that intrinsic muscle function alone is enough to extend the IP joints

EDM: ask the patient to make a fist and only extend the little finger in the MCP joint.

ECU: ask the patient to extend the wrist and deviate ulnar.

INTRINSIC MUSCLES

THENAR MUSCLES

APB, OP and FPB: together these provide pronation and opposition of the thumb. Ask the patient to place the tip of the thumb against the tip of the little finger (forming an 'O'), with the nails in the same plane (opposition). Ask the patient to position their hand flat on the table palm up and then lift the extended thumb (palmar abduction) (Figure 3.4).

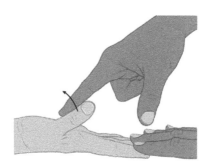

Figure 3.4 Examination of the m. abductor pollicis brevis (median nerve).

AdP: allow the patient to hold a piece of paper between the tip of the stretched thumb and the radial side of the index finger. In case of failure of the m. adductor pollicis (generally due to ulnar nerve injury) the patient will flex the IP joint of the thumb to be able to hold the paper. This is Froment's sign.

Mm. interossei and mm. lumbricales: these flex the MCP joint and extend the PIP joint. The mm. interossei also abduct (dorsal mm. interossei) and adduct (volar mm. interossei) the fingers.

Hypothenar

ADM, FDM and ODM: these are tested as a group. Ask the patient to position the hand flat on the table palm down and abduct the little finger. Palpate the muscle belly on the ulnar side of the palm.

NERVES

If a nerve injury is suspected, the muscles and skin it innervates are examined. The median nerve and the ulnar nerve are mixed nerves at the level of the wrist, meaning they have both a motor and sensory function. With injury of sensory nerves, there will be numbness distal to the trauma. Additionally, the skin becomes dry and can feel smoother due to decreased sweat secretion.

Sensibility can be tested by comparing it with a non-affected finger. This can be tested by lightly stroking the affected area with your fingertip and have the patient compare it to a similar non-affected area. If the patient notes a difference, often indicated as 'different', 'less', or 'numb', nerve injury should be excluded. Do not test sensibility with needle pricks: you only have to stimulate one intact axon to falsely conclude no nerve injury. A more sensitive way is to use a bent paperclip to determine two-point discrimination (2PD). One or two ends are pressed longitudinal to each other on one side of the finger until blanching occurs. The patient should be able to distinguish one or two ends.

You can bring the ends further apart until two-point discrimination is noted. A normal 2PD in a fingertip is 4–6 mm.

BLOOD VESSELS

Congested (problem with venous outflow): blue discoloration, accelerated capillary refill, swelling.

Absent or reduced arterial supply: pale, diminished turgor, delayed capillary refill, lower temperature.

Test for arterial flow (capillary refill): press the nail; a pink colour should return in less than two seconds after pressure is removed.

Pulse: palpate the radial artery and ulnar artery. Although not very sensitive (due to an incomplete vascular arch or a significant median artery), the Allen test can provide a rough estimation of the patency. The test is performed by asking a patient to clench their fist several times while the examiner occludes the radial and ulnar artery by applying pressure. The patient then extends their fingers, showing a blanched hand, while still applying pressure. By lifting the compression on one of the arteries, its patency can be assessed.

BONES

INSPECTION

Look for abnormal positions and rotational deformities.

PALPATION

The classic fracture symptom, pain on axial compression, is often not present in hand fractures (condylar fractures, avulsion fractures). Pain on palpation is present. Crepitation should not be actively searched for in case a fracture is suspected.

PHYSICAL EXAMINATION

Swelling limits the mobility of the joints. The 'range of motion' (ROM) decreases compared with the non-affected side. Pain can also be the cause of loss of motion.

In case a fracture or luxation is suspected, it is wise to first perform X-ray examination. Stability of joints can be assessed by 'stressing' the joint and comparing it with the contralateral (healthy) side. The IP joints of the fingers and the MCP joint of the thumb are stable in extension. The MCP joints of the fingers are stable in flexion.

4

Imaging

X-rays are requested following a clinical suspicion, where the image serves to confirm the diagnosis. Always judge the image yourself. When requesting X-ray images, make sure to specify the clinical findings and suspicion, the area to be imaged and, if applicable, non-routine views. Some fractures of the carpal bones can only become visible with special views (i.e. carpal tunnel view for fractures of the hook of hamate, Bett's view for a clear view of the CMC1 joint).

The technician will use the appropriate technique if the request is done clearly. A CT scan is indicated in case of comminuted intra-articular fractures, scaphoid fractures or to assess complex luxations. Ultrasound is a suitable medium for demonstrating foreign bodies. Arthroscopy can be used in the acute stage to help in the reduction of intra-articular radial fractures. The knowledge of surface anatomy related to the X-ray image is important (Figures 4.1–4.5).

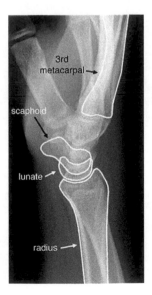

Figure 4.1 Lateral view of the wrist.

DOI: 10.1201/9781003313540-4

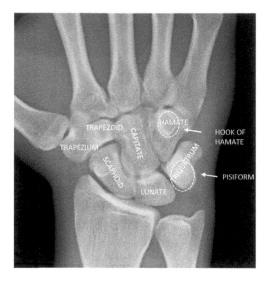

Figure 4.2 Carpal bones.

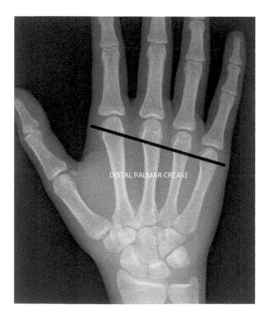

Figure 4.3 Distal palmar crease, position of the MCP joints.

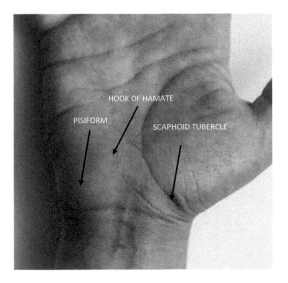

Figure 4.4 Anatomy landmarks in the palm of the hand.

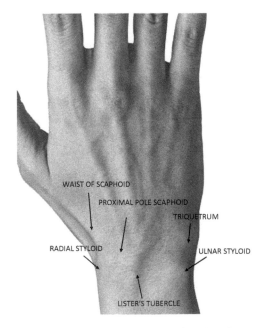

Figure 4.5 Anatomy landmarks of the dorsum of the hand.

5

Anesthesia

GENERAL

First investigate, then anesthetize!

Small procedures may be performed under local anesthesia. In other cases regional or general anesthesia is used. Contrary to common belief, local anesthetic with adrenaline can safely be used in the extremity of healthy patients. It was previously believed that adrenaline would cause spasm of the terminal arteries and cause necrosis. This is not true. A so-called Bier's block is less suitable for hand surgery. The possible operating time is short, no longer than one hour. Additionally, when the tourniquet is released, there is no longer any possibility of performing hemostasis.

The most commonly used local anesthetic is lidocaine. The maximum dose of lidocaine with adrenaline (1:100,000) is 7 mg/kg body weight. [25 mL 2% solution, or 50 mL 1% solution]. Warming the anesthetic to body temperature and adding sodium bicarbonate 8.4% (in a ratio of 1:10 in case of a 1% lidocaine with 1:100,000 adrenaline) makes the injection substantially less painful.

LOCAL ANESTHESIA

In case of lacerations, the wound edges are injected. A needle can also be used directly in the wound. Do not anesthetize a fingertip by directly injecting into the pulp – this is extremely painful. A finger can be easily anesthetized through an Oberst's anesthesia (Figure 5.1). Inject dorsally or volarly, just proximal to the middle of the proximal phalanges. Deposit a small amount of approximately 2 mL on both sides on the volar aspect (Figure 5.1). The thumb can also be anesthetized by means of Oberst's anesthesia, but the dorsal site must also be injected due to a separate nerve innervation. A bloodless field can be created by applying a small tourniquet on the finger proximally with a silicone drain. Place a clamp on the drain such that the drain does not accidentally disappear under the dressing!

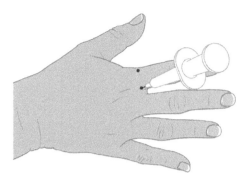

Figure 5.1 Oberst's anesthesia.

REGIONAL ANESTHESIA

Conduction anesthesia in the form of a brachial plexus block is performed by experienced anesthetists or hand surgeons. Generating paresthesia at a peripheral nerve with an ordinary hypodermic needle is undesirable because it can cause nerve damage.

MEDIAN NERVE BLOCK AT THE LEVEL OF THE WRIST

Inject one to two centimeters in the carpal tunnel proximal to the wrist fold between the FCR and the PL. A bolus of a few milliliters is sufficient. If no sign of paresthesia occurs after five minutes, the procedure may be repeated.

ULNAR NERVE BLOCK AT THE LEVEL OF THE WRIST

Inject radial to the FCU tendon, just below the tendon and proximal to the os pisiforme. As always, aspirate before injecting as the ulnar artery is nearby.

ULNAR NERVE BLOCK AT THE LEVEL OF THE ELBOW

Inject at the proximal end of the fossa olecrani.

RADIAL NERVE BLOCK AT THE LEVEL OF THE WRIST

Inject a bolus on the radial side of the wrist, from volar to dorsal, a few centimeters proximal to the anatomical snuff box. It hereby blocks all branches of the superficial radial nerve.

Intoxications in the use of anesthetics may occur due to the use of excessive quantity or concentration, or by intravascular injection.

TOURNIQUET-INDUCED EXSANGUINATION

For the upper extremity, a tourniquet cuff can be used. As mentioned before, a silicone drain can be used for a finger. The use of a piece of a glove and rolling it down the patient's finger is dangerous when forgetting to remove it before applying a bandage.

TECHNIQUE

Wrap a thin layer of cotton wool around the upper arm. Apply the tourniquet such that it is snug – if it is too tight it causes venous congestion. Elevate the arm and inflate the cuff quickly, preferably to 70–100 mm of mercury above the patient's systolic blood pressure. Always note the starting time, as the tourniquet time should last no longer than two hours. If two hours are reached, the tourniquet must be released for a minimum of 15 minutes before re-application. The cuff can only be tolerated for a maximum of 10–20 minutes without anesthesia. Known complications are nerve damage due to excessive pressure or prolonged compression, and chemical burns due to disinfectants underneath the cuff. Exsanguination with Esmarch or Martin bandage are optional, but should not be used in case of an infection, a ganglion or a malignant tumor.

6

Soft tissue injuries

The objective of treatment is to maintain or create durable soft tissue coverage, allowing optimal function and sensibility. A thorough debridement of avascular or bruised tissue is essential. After this, a wound can be closed taking the following into account:

- A wound can be primarily closed if there is no tension on the wound edges while doing so. In all other cases, a consultation by a hand surgeon is required.
- In the event of a skin shortage and a well vascularized wound surface, the defect can be closed with a full or partial thickness skin graft.
- Donor sites for a partial thickness graft in order of preference are: medial side of the leg, buttock, abdomen, medial side upper arm and skull. For small defects the hypothenar skin graft is very suitable. Donor sites for full thickness grafts in order of preference are: groin, medial side upper arm, retro- or pre-auricular, supraclavicular and, if possible, upper eyelid.
- In case of skin shortage and visible 'white structures' (i.e. bone, tendon, ligament, nerve), closure of the defect with a skin graft is no longer possible.
- The defect should be closed with a local transposition flap or a free vascularized flap. The exception being extensor tendons – if they are still covered with paratenon (the areolar tissue which allows gliding of the tendon), they can be covered with a skin graft.
- In case of avulsion injuries, the tissue's vascularization is often overestimated. In most cases it is wise to obtain a skin graft from the avulsed flap and use that as coverage.
- In case of a deficit of the fingers it is important whether there is loss of pulp, exposed extensor or flexor tendons and/or a defect in a functional area. If a skin graft is applied, it should be full thickness to prevent contracture and supply a more durable surface.
- If closure of a small defect is not possible with a skin graft many local transposition flaps are available. For larger skin defects, particularly on the back of the hand, it is possible to use a pedicled flap or a free vascularized lap.

DOI: 10.1201/9781003313540-6

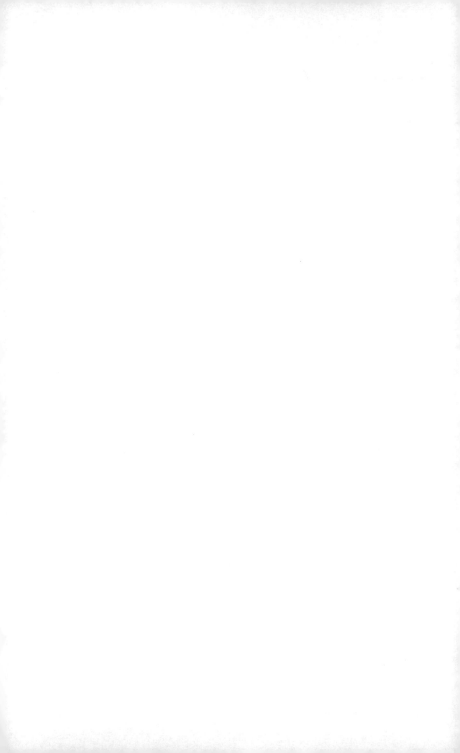

Extensor tendon injuries

MALLET FINGER

PATIENT HISTORY

A sudden flexion force in a stretched finger causes a closed extensor tendon rupture at the DIP joint. This often occurs when making a bed, or during ball games in young patients ('baseball finger'). In the latter case an avulsion fracture is possible.

PHYSICAL EXAMINATION

Full active extension of the DIP joint is not possible. Full passive extension is possible. If the injury has occurred during ball sports or by any other strong force, there is an indication for an X-ray to diagnose a possible bony avulsion.

TREATMENT

With a closed rupture, with or without a small bone fragment (less than one third of the joint surface and no significant volar subluxation of the distal phalanx), a conservative treatment is sufficient for approximately 60% of cases with a so-called Stack (or Stax) splint (Figure 7.1). This splint immobilizes the DIP joint in slight hyperextension for six to eight weeks.

The splint should be worn 24 hours a day. The PIP joint remains free to allow flexion. In patients who do not adhere to therapy a trans-articular Kirschner wire can be chosen for fixation. With an open mallet finger or with an avulsion fragment larger than one third of the joint surface or in cases of subluxation of the distal phalanx, operative repair is indicated.

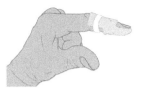

Figure 7.1 Stack splint. The PIP joint remains free.

PROGNOSIS

After treatment with a Stack splint, it is sometimes necessary to continue the treatment for a prolonged period if the patient is willing to. Ultimately, further recovery can occur in the course of one year. An extension deficit of less than 20° is not considered functionally disabling and does not require treatment. In a chronic mallet finger, a hyperextension of the PIP joint can occur, causing the finger to have a swan neck deformity.

BOUTONNIÈRE DEFORMITY

PATIENT HISTORY

This is a closed or open avulsion injury of the central slip of the extensor aponeurosis at the PIP joint. The injury often occurs after a volar luxation of the PIP joint. This injury is often missed at presentation, as initially complete extension is still possible. After several days gradual volar sliding of the lateral slips occurs, creating the typical Boutonnière deformity (Figure 7.2).

EXAMINATION

In the acute phase, the patient experiences pain at the level of the PIP joint. In a closed rupture there is swelling on the dorsal side where sometimes the avulsed central slip is palpable. If examined carefully, a slight extension deficit is noted. The Elson test is performed; ask the patient to bend the PIP joint 90° over the edge of the table and extend the middle phalanx against resistance. In presence of central slip injury there will be a weak PIP extension and a rigid DIP (due

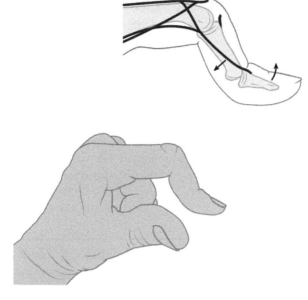

Figure 7.2 Boutonnière deformity.

to pulling of the lateral slips). Closed injury require X-ray investigation in two directions to exclude an avulsion fracture.

TREATMENT

A closed injury is treated with a splint with the PIP joint immobilized in extension for six weeks. The other finger joints have free range of motion. An open injury is treated by tendon repair or reinsertion and immobilization by means of a trans-articular Kirschner wire.

PROGNOSIS

In most cases, this tendon injury is only recognized after a Boutonnière deformity has established. The late correction of a Boutonnière deformity is often a disappointing procedure which rarely leads to good results.

EXTENSOR TENDON INJURY AT THE LEVEL OF THE MCP JOINTS AND THE DORSUM OF THE HAND

PATIENT HISTORY

Extensor tendon injury at the level of the MCP joints is often caused by bite injuries as a result of a punch. The risk of a septic arthritis of the MCP joint is high. Spontaneous ruptures of extensor tendons are possible due to rheumatoid arthritis and fractures (i.e. distal radius fracture followed by an EPL rupture).

Sometimes an acute compression of the dorsal interosseus nerve can lead to inability to extend the MP joint.

EXAMINATION

In case of a laceration at MCP level, there is initially only a small extension deficit because of the juncturae tendinum. Inspect the finger cascade. Don't be fooled – the IP joints of the fingers can be fully extended by the intrinsic musculature despite a transection of the long extensor tendon! More specifically examine the independent extension of the index finger to establish a transection of the EIP tendon. X-ray imaging is indicated in case of tendon injury by a foreign body such as glass or teeth.

TREATMENT

Extensor tendon ruptures are sutured with horizontal mattress sutures. If the dorsal skin covering the tendon is thin, it is best to use an a-traumatic absorbable 4-0 suture. A monofilament 6-0 can be used for additional adjustments. Repair of lacerations of the extensor hood over the fingers is reserved for a hand surgeon.

At the level of the back of the hand extensor tendons can be sutured under local anesthesia. Retrieval of an EPL tendon sectioned at the level of the first metacarpal is only possible with regional or general anesthesia. The aftertreatment is usually static but a dynamic aftertreatment may be indicated.

A volar plaster splint is applied with the wrist in 40° extension, MCP joints in 30° flexion and the IP joints in neutral position ('position of protection'). Remove the splint and skin stitches after four weeks and start hand therapy. After repair of EDCs it is justified to exclude the PIP joints from the plaster.

Flexor tendon and nerve injuries

8

INTRODUCTION

Most flexor tendon and nerve injuries are caused by a glass or knife injury to the volar side of the hand. An open flexor tendon injury is often accompanied by nerve injury.

PHYSICAL EXAMINATION

Examine the individual flexor tendons. Examine the target area of the nerve that may be intersected. Test the sensibility of both the ulnar and radial side of the injured finger. Compare this with a non-affected side. In children one can stroke the finger with a pen. After nerve transection, sweat secretion is diminished and the skin feels smoother. In case of injuries in the palm of the hand or in the forearm the motor function of the nerves should also tested. A change in nerve function does not necessarily mean that the continuity of the nerve is lost – there may be neurapraxia. Suppress the tendency to place clamps or sutures in the wound; this makes recovery of nerve and vascular injury more difficult. An often-missed injury is the closed avulsion of the FDP tendon of the distal phalanx ('Jersey finger'). X-ray imaging does not always show an osseous avulsion fragment.

IMAGING

In case of sharp lacerations no additional imaging is required. In case of crush injury and/or a suspicion of a tendon avulsion an X-ray in PA and lateral direction should be obtained.

DOI: 10.1201/9781003313540-8

TREATMENT

In the event of any suspicion of a flexor tendon or nerve injury, a hand surgeon must be consulted. Do not explore the wound and certainly do not place any form of suture or clamps in the wound. Do not anesthetize the finger because this hinders the examination of sensibility. If direct treatment is not possible, flush the wound with copious saline and leave the wound open.

Nerve injuries should be repaired with microsurgical techniques and magnification. Although not all nerve injuries are repaired, this is a decision that must be taken by the hand surgeon on the basis of a number of factors: which nerve, which finger, which hand, and the age and profession of the patient.

Nerve repair will not always lead to complete recovery, but it can prevent the development of painful neuromas.

Postoperative rehabilitation is very important.

9

Fingertip injury

PATIENT HISTORY

Ask about the nature of the injury. Factors such as age, profession, hobbies, affected finger and hand-dominance are important.

PHYSICAL EXAMINATION

As mentioned earlier, the location is important. In addition, exposed bone affects the treatment chosen. The exact depth and surface area are assessed after debridement.

TREATMENT

Small injuries of the fingertip, especially in children, can be treated conservatively. Shortening of the bone is rarely necessary. Injuries with a surface area of more than 1 cm² and intact pulp can be closed with a skin graft. Skin grafts of full thickness are preferred to prevent contraction. Preferable donor sites are the amputated part itself, the hypothenar area, and for larger areas in order of preference the groin, medial upper arm and elbow crease.

In case of exposed bone a local transposition flap is required. This type of reconstruction belongs in the armamentarium of hand surgeons. Fingertip injuries involving the nail complex should have the subungual hematoma drained by drilling a small hole in the nail plate (or puncturing it with a heated paperclip). A subungual hematoma covering more than 50% of the surface area requires removal of the nail and repairing the nail bed with 6-0 absorbable sutures. The eponychium is kept open by replacing the old nail. In case of defects of the nail bed, a nail bed graft may be considered. This too belongs to the area of the hand surgeon.

Tip lesions with a fracture of the distal phalanx, if not intra-articular, can be treated conservatively.

10

Luxations of the fingers and midhand

DIP JOINT

INTRODUCTION

This luxation is rare and usually to dorsal or lateral. Often it is an open injury (Figure 10.1).

PATIENT HISTORY

More often than not, the luxation will have already been repositioned by the patient.

PHYSICAL EXAMINATION

Test stability and exclude soft tissue interposition. Test the passive mobility of the joint. In children, an open physeal fracture of the distal phalanx can occur with interposition of the nail wall (Seymour fracture).

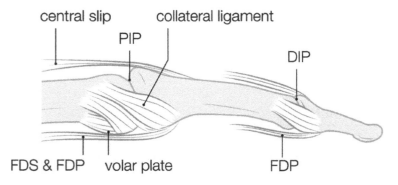

Figure 10.1 Ligaments of the IP joints.

DOI: 10.1201/9781003313540-10

IMAGING

X-rays in PA and lateral direction before and after reposition.

TREATMENT

With a stable joint after reposition, three weeks of plaster enclosing the DIP joint is sufficient. Larger avulsion fragments and instabilities require surgery.

Seymour lesions require surgical treatment.

PIP JOINT

INTRODUCTION

A dorsal luxation of the PIP joint can cause damage to the volar plate and collateral ligaments. The luxation can be open. Untreated subluxation leads to chronic instability and/or a swan neck deformity.

ANAMNESIS

Often the PIP was forced in hyperextension by a ball or a fall. It usually concerns the index or ring finger.

IMAGING

X-rays in PA and lateral direction to exclude avulsion fractures.

TREATMENT

If the joint is stable after repositioning, an extension-blocking splint is sufficient. Surgical treatment is indicated in the event of instability, interposition, a wound on the volar side of the joint or an avulsion fragment larger than 30% of the joint surface.

MCP JOINT

INTRODUCTION

MCP luxations are most common in the thumb. It usually involves the ulnar collateral ligament (UCL), sometimes in combination with a volar plate avulsion. This 'skier's thumb' is not the same as a 'gamekeeper's thumb'. The former concerns a rupture of the ulnar collateral ligament, while the latter involves a stretching of the ligament due to repetitive movements. A so-called Stener lesion indicates there is a complete rupture of the ulnar collateral ligament in which the aponeurosis of the m. adductor pollicis is interposed between the UCL and its insertion to the proximal phalanx. Conservative treatment is therefore not possible. The MCP joints of the fingers have a possibility of a dorsal luxation, whereby the head of the os metacarpal is fixed between the flexor tendons, the volar plate and the intrinsic musculature. This requires an open reposition.

PATIENT HISTORY

The trauma mechanism is important to be able to determine which ligament is damaged.

PHYSICAL EXAMINATION

Determine the point of maximal swelling and pain on palpation. Stress the joint, if necessary after anesthesia, in 0° and 30° of flexion to establish instability.

IMAGING

Request X-ray images in AP and lateral direction to exclude avulsions. Ultrasound can detect a Stener lesion in experienced hands.

TREATMENT

In the event of a distortion (partial rupture) of the ulnar collateral ligament: two weeks of plaster immobilization, followed by four weeks of tape treatment. A complete rupture of the ulnar collateral ligament is an indication for operative repair. If the rupture involves an avulsion without displacement four weeks immobilization will suffice.

Carpal luxations

INTRODUCTION

Seven per cent of all carpal injuries are dislocations of the carpus with or without a fracture. These injuries are often primarily missed.

Os lunatum luxations

It usually involves a volar luxation (Figure 11.1). X-ray imaging in AP direction will show minimal deviations in the carpus, but lateral views clearly show the extent of the luxation. The treatment in the acute stage consists of open reposition and ligament repair.

PERILUNATE DISLOCATIONS

Introduction

The mechanism of injury often involves a traumatic hyperextension and ulnar deviation of the wrist leading to a rupture of the scapholunate (Figure 11.2) (SL) and lunotriquetral (LT) ligaments (Figure 11.3). The perilunate dislocation can be pure ligamentous or in combination with a fracture, in which the scaphoid is most commonly affected (Figure 11.3).

Physical examination

In a perilunate fracture-dislocation, the severity of the injury is often not visible externally. Patients experience diffuse swelling and pain, with a painful limited motion of the wrist. The sensibility in the median nerve and ulnar nerve distribution is disturbed. On palpation, the dorsal dislocation of the os capitatum can be felt.

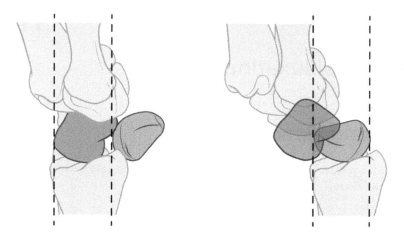

Figure 11.1 Left: volar lunate luxation. Right: dorsal perilunate dislocation.

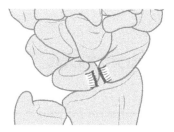

Figure 11.2 SL ligament rupture.

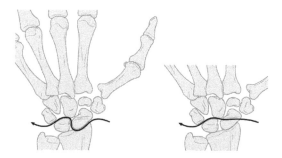

Figure 11.3 Left: rupture of SL and LT ligament. Right: fracture of the scaphoid and rupture of LT ligament.

IMAGING

Usually a PA and lateral X-ray of the wrist are sufficient. In case a scaphoid fracture is suspected, additional scaphoid series should be requested.

Approximately 20% of perilunate dislocations are missed on the initial X-ray. Assess the contours and position of the carpal bones and compare with the contralateral healthy side. Review the lines of Gilula for disfigurements (Figure 11.4). A CT scan is commonly obtained.

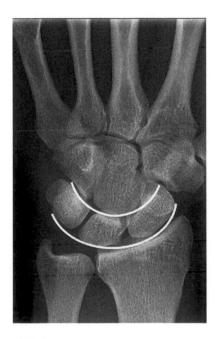

Figure 11.4 Lines of Gilula.

Fractures of the hand

POINT OF ATTENTION

Improper treatment can lead to significant loss of function and possibly the inability to work.

GENERAL

Fractures of phalanges and metacarpals are the most common fractures seen in the Emergency Department. The treatment focuses on anatomical reposition and early mobilization, possibly under the supervision of a hand therapist. Spiral fractures bear the risk of rotational deformities. Oblique and comminuted fractures can cause shortening and angulation deformities. Avulsion fractures at the base of the phalanges can be an indication of more complex injuries.

PHYSICAL EXAMINATION

Classic symptoms can be absent in hand fractures. Crepitus or instability can be seen with unintended manipulation. Rotational deformities can be detected by flexion of the MCP joints to 90° and the IP joints stretched. In this position, the nails should align almost parallel. With the MCP and PIP joints flexed (and the DIP extended), the fingertips should all point to just proximal of the scaphoid tubercle (Figure 12.1).

IMAGING

X-rays in PA and lateral direction, and a ¾ view for IP joint fractures.

DESCRIBING THE FRACTURE

Fracture type: avulsion/transverse/spiral/oblique/comminuted

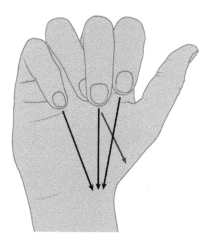

Figure 12.1 Flexion of MCP and PIP joints should have all nails pointing towards the scaphoid tubercle.

Location: intra/extra-articular/tuft/base/shaft/sub capital/caput
Position: dislocated/non-dislocated
Open or closed

NON-SURGICAL TREATMENT

Indications for conservative treatment are:

- extra-articular, non-dislocated transverse or oblique fractures
- dislocated fractures that are stable after repositioning. The reposition must remain stable in a plaster splint in 'intrinsic plus' position. Prolonged immobilization in any other position may lead to contractures.

Non-dislocated stable fractures can sometimes be treated by means of 'buddy taping' to the adjacent finger during two to three weeks. However, the intrinsic and extrinsic tendons can cause a secondary dislocation. Therefore position must be checked with X-ray imaging after one week.

SURGICAL TREATMENT

In general, any fracture that remains unstable in an 'intrinsic plus' position requires surgery. Other indications for surgery are intra-articular fractures, spiral or comminuted fractures, oblique fractures with shortening, and open fractures in combination with soft tissue injuries (especially tendon or neuro-vascular injury).

Surgical treatment may consist of:

- closed reduction and percutaneous osteosynthesis
- open reduction and osteosynthesis
- dynamic traction
- external fixation

FRACTURES IN CHILDREN

The growth plates of the phalanges are located at the proximal end. Epiphyseal fractures can be classified according to Salter and Harris (Figure 12.2). A deviation of less than ten degrees is acceptable when the fracture is located at the base of the proximal phalanx. Deviations are not acceptable in the middle and distal phalanx as the natural correction during growth in these phalanges is minimal.

Dislocated epiphyseal fractures of the proximal phalanges Salter Harris types I and II can often be repositioned with a ballpoint pen in the digital web as a lever. In case of Salter Harris types III, IV and V fractures, consult a hand surgeon. The open epiphyseal fracture of the distal phalanx is often not recognized. There may be interposition of the nail bed (Seymour lesion).

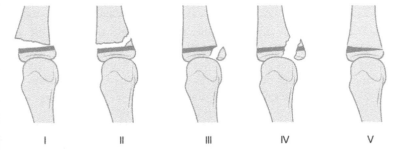

Figure 12.2 Salter-Harris classification of epiphyseal fractures.

SPECIAL FRACTURES

CONDYLAR FRACTURES

Condylar fractures of the phalanx are underestimated in terms of severity. Perfect repositioning is a prerequisite for a functional IP joint.

AVULSION FRACTURES

Avulsion fragments can be a sign of avulsion of the extensor tendon, the flexor tendon, the volar plate or the collateral ligaments. A mallet fracture is an avulsion of the insertion of the extensor tendon on the dorsal side onto the base of the distal phalanx. It is treated with a short extension splint, also called mallet or Stack splint for a minimum of four to six weeks. The PIP joint must be free to flex and extend in the splint. If the avulsion entails more than one third of the base of the distal phalanx surgical treatment is often preferred. For certain when there is a volar subluxation of the distal phalanx.

METACARPAL FRACTURES

POINT OF ATTENTION

In the case of fractures at the base of the metacarpal bone, dislocation of the carpo-metacarpal joint should be excluded.

GENERAL

The fracture is usually caused by a direct trauma. Metacarpal II and III are rigidly fixed to the carpus, metacarpal IV and V have a greater mobility. This allows for more tolerance for angulation of fractures of metacarpal IV and V. Rotational errors must be corrected. These are mainly seen in metacarpal II and V because the intermetacarpal ligament is present on one side only.

PHYSICAL EXAMINATION

Typical symptoms include swelling, pain and sometimes loss of height of the knuckle (flattening of the metacarpal arch). Sometimes crepitus or instability during manipulation is present. Pay attention to any rotational deformity of the finger. A five degree rotational deformity of the metacarpal will result in a 1.5 centimeter overlap at the level of distal phalanx during flexion.

IMAGING

X-rays in AP and lateral direction, and ¾ if deemed necessary.

CONSERVATIVE TREATMENT

A single transverse or oblique fracture can be treated conservatively if it is stable after reduction. Rotational deformities may not be accepted.

For the second and third metacarpal, an angulation of ten degrees maximum is acceptable. For the fourth and fifth metacarpal this is 20° and 30° respectively. In fifth metacarpal neck fractures ('boxer's fracture'), a dorsal angulation up to 40° is acceptable. Treatment, after closed reduction, generally consists of a plaster splint up to the PIP joints with the MCP joints flexed and the wrist joint in 20° extension for four weeks. There are advocates for a functional rehabilitation in a pressure bandage, especially in weekend recidivists.

SURGICAL TREATMENT

Surgical treatment follows after consultation with a hand surgeon. This is recommended for spiral or oblique fractures with a rotational deformity, comminuted fractures, open fractures, unstable fractures, and intra-articular luxation fractures of the CMC joints.

The surgical treatment may consist of:

- closed reduction and percutaneous fixation
- open reduction and osteosynthesis
- external fixation

SPECIAL FRACTURES

BENNETT FRACTURE

This is an intra-articular, single fragment fracture of the base of the first metacarpal. Because of traction of the m. abductor pollicis longus, the base

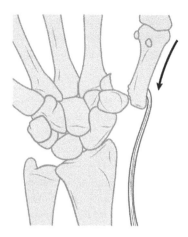

Figure 12.3 Bennett fracture.

of the metacarpal migrates proximally. Treatment is almost always surgical (Figure 12.3).

REVERSED BENNETT FRACTURE

This consists of an intra-articular fracture at the base of the fifth metacarpal. Traction of the m. extensor carpi ulnaris pulls the base of metacarpal proximally. Like a regular Bennett fracture, treatment is almost always surgical.

ROLANDO FRACTURE

Any comminuted intra-articular fracture of the base of the first metacarpal is a Rolando fracture. The treatment is almost always surgical.

SCAPHOID FRACTURES

POINTS OF ATTENTION

This is an often-missed fracture. Postponement of treatment may lead to a delayed union, malunion or non-union. This fracture can be part of a distal radius fracture or more complex luxation fractures of the carpus.

PATIENT HISTORY

This fracture often occurs in young men and rarely in children. In most cases there is a fall on the outstretched hand (FOOSH) or a punch with a clenched fist.

PHYSICAL EXAMINATION

Typical symptoms include a pronounced swelling and pain on palpation in the anatomical snuff box. Sometimes there is swelling of the entire wrist, which makes the pain difficult to localize.

IMAGING

X-rays in PA and lateral direction. In case of a strong clinical suspicion this can be supplemented with PA radiographs with the wrist in ulnar and radial deviation. Further additional imaging such as a bone, CT or MRI scan can be requested on indication.

TREATMENT

Stable, non-dislocated fractures are treated with immobilization. Stable fractures are incomplete fractures or fractures of the distal pole tubercle.

A distal pole fracture needs eight weeks immobilization. Non-stable or dislocated fractures are treated with open fixation with specially developed screws.

FOLLOW-UP

If there is a strong clinical suspicion of a scaphoid fracture, but there is no clear fracture visible on the initial X-ray, then the wrist should be immobilized and physical examination and X-rays repeated after two weeks. A CT scan can be a superior option.

PROGNOSIS

Appropriate treatment leads to consolidation in 90% of cases. In case of non-union, and in particular osteonecrosis of the proximal pole, surgical treatment is required to prevent further degenerative changes.

DISTAL RADIUS FRACTURE

POINTS OF ATTENTION

This is a very common fracture (15% of all fractures). There are two incidence peaks, namely at a young age and between the ages of 60 and 70.

PATIENT HISTORY

In most cases there has been a FOOSH. Other mechanisms are possible, leading to a multiplicity of fracture types.

PHYSICAL EXAMINATION

There is a swelling of the wrist, accompanied with pain. Sometimes there is a visible deformation. Also pay attention to accompanying injuries to the elbow or shoulder.

IMAGING

X-rays in PA and lateral direction. Note the length of the radius, the radial inclination and volar tilting of the joint surface, intra-articular fractures of the radius or DRU joint, and any fracture of the ulnar styloid (TFC involvement). If indicated, take X-rays of the entire forearm. In case of a complex comminuted or intra-articular fractures, there may be an indication for a CT scan.

TREATMENT

Treatment is aimed at restoring normal anatomy, taking into account the age of the patient and his/her requirements and needs.

In the case of an isolated fracture of the ulnar styloid, the arm is immobilized for three weeks in an upper arm cast. If the fracture is located at the base of the styloid with a dislocation of more than 5 mm and a widened DRU joint, then surgical fixation is indicated to fix an avulsed TFC ligament.

Non-displaced fractures, whether intra- or extra-articular, can be treated by immobilization for six weeks. A follow-up X-ray is obtained after one week to rule out dislocation.

Displaced fractures, both extra- and intra-articular, can sometimes be treated conservatively after reduction in traction.

If the position is unstable or there is gross dislocation of fragments with shortening, operative fixation is indicated with percutaneous K-wire fixation, open reduction and internal fixation, external fixation or a combination of these options.

POST-TREATMENT

Plaster immobilization should allow room for swelling, especially in the first week. Compression leads to carpal tunnel syndrome and/or a higher incidence of CRPS. After one week, the plaster is replaced and X-rays are taken in two directions in the new plaster. The total immobilization should last five to six weeks. If the reposition is lost, surgical intervention can still be planned.

PROGNOSIS

Non-union seldom occurs. A malunion (i.e., an inverted joint plane and/or a shortening) can cause a secondary collapse of the carpal bones. In the event of a serious shortening, patients can experience complaints due to a relatively long ulna and/or DRU joint incongruence. Pain (especially in combination with swelling of the fingers) is always a reason to see the patient again. The plaster or splint must be completely removed. One should be aware of a carpal tunnel syndrome. A rupture of the EPL tendon is sometimes an additional (late) complication of a conservative treatment.

13

Amputations and ring avulsions

AMPUTATIONS

POINTS OF ATTENTION

Avoid delay and damage to the stump and/or amputate. Cool the amputated finger, but never put it directly on ice. The amputated part should be wrapped in a moist gauze and placed in a sealable plastic bag, which is then put on ice.

There is an absolute indication for replantation in the following:

- children
- amputation of the thumb
- amputation of multiple fingers
- amputation level through the palm, wrist or forearm

Indication for replantation of a single finger may be:

- amputation in children
- sharp, distal amputation beyond the FDS insertion (zone I)
- individual requirements

PHYSICAL EXAMINATION

Determine the level and extent of the amputation and the amount of soft tissue damage. In a partial amputation, the distal circulation, sensibility and function are tested.

IMAGING

X-ray examination of the stump and amputate.

DOI: 10.1201/9781003313540-13

TREATMENT

Factors that influence the outcome are the extent of crush injury to the blood vessels, whether the patient is a smoker, and the total ischemia time. A replantation should always be performed by an experienced hand surgeon. An honest discussion about the functional result of an replantation is warranted.

RING AVULSIONS

POINTS OF ATTENTION

Remove the ring. The ring may be hidden underneath the skin and subcutis.

Examination of vascularization is difficult. Avulsed soft tissue with some circulation can look deceptively good at first glance. Length of ischemia is the most important factor in determining outcome.

PHYSICAL EXAMINATION

Which structures are avulsed? Are the neurovascular bundles intact? Make a distinction between normal circulation, no vascular filling with low turgor, and venous congestion. Test the sensibility. Test flexion and extension.

X-ray in PA and lateral direction to diagnose or rule out fractures.

TREATMENT

Remove the ring. If no skin defect or only a laceration is present, the vascularization and sensitivity are normal, and there is a normal function and no fracture, the patient should start with early mobilization.

In all other cases, a hand surgeon should assess the finger.

FOLLOW-UP

Inspection after 24 hours. Explain to the patient that when in doubt, he or she should return sooner.

14

Hand infections

FELON INFECTION

GENERAL

This is a deep infection in the closed space of the soft tissues of a fingertip usually caused by a Staphylococcus aureus.

The infection evolves, often after a minimal trauma, in two to five days into an abscess with increasing pain.

TREATMENT

First, the exact location of the felon is determined. Let the patient identify the point of maximum tenderness. After anesthesia (Oberst) and with a finger tourniquet, an ellipse-shaped excision is performed at the site of maximum pain. The cavity is opened and rinsed, and necrosis removed. The incision is left open and inspected daily. Antibiotics are not indicated in this stage.

Fish-mouth incisions, 'hockey stick' incision and through-and-through incisions are obsolete.

PARONYCHIA

GENERAL

This is an infection of the skin around the nail, usually the cuticle.

POINTS OF ATTENTION

In the acute phase, inadequate recognition or therapy can lead to a pulp infection (felon) or a flexor sheath infection.

The cause of the infection is usually a Staphylococcus aureus.

TREATMENT

At the onset of redness, oral antibiotics can still be effective.

In case of abscess formation, drainage after removing a small longitudinal part of the nail under Oberst anesthesia is necessary.

In all cases, consider the possibility of a candida albicans or herpes infection, or malignancy.

ERYSIPELAS

GENERAL

This is a streptococcus infection of the skin and subcutaneous tissue.

PATIENT HISTORY

The infection is usually caused by a minor trauma, such as a puncture wound or small breakage of the skin, and can become fulminant within 6–36 hours.

There is a swelling and redness of the hand, sometimes accompanied by ascending lymphangitis and lymphadenitis.

TREATMENT

Treatment should consist of a high dose of a penicillin derivative intravenously. It is strongly advised to mark the redness pre-treatment, so that the evolution of the infection can be followed. Surgical exploration is pointless. Patient or doctor's delay can lead to necrotizing fasciitis.

BITE WOUNDS INFECTIONS

GENERAL

Cat bites can cause severe necrotizing infection (Pasteurella multocida). Do not miss the small wounds, usually at the level of MCP III, IV or V, after a punch in which a human tooth of the opponent has opened the joint. Human bites often cause hemolytic streptococcus, staphylococcus aureus or eikenella corrodens infections. An X-ray is required to detect a fracture and/or a foreign body.

TREATMENT

Debride and rinse with saline. Leave the wound open. Administer the patient intravenous antibiotics, and elevate and immobilize the hand. The choice of the antibiotic should be consulted with the microbiologist.

FLEXOR SHEATH INFECTION

GENERAL

Early recognition of an infection of the tendon sheath prevents a potential necrotic tendon or more proximal spread of the infection (phlegmon).

SYMPTOMS

Look for the four 'cardinal' signs of Kanavel: flexed posture of the involved finger, fusiform swelling, pain with active and passive extension, painful palpation of the tendon sheath (up to the palm).

TREATMENT BY HAND SURGEON

The tendon sheath must be explored urgently. The tendon sheath is opened proximally at the A1-pulley level and distally at the level of the A5 pulley/DIP joint. With a small catheter the sheath is rinsed with saline. **Do not close the incisions!** A permanent flushing system is not indicated. The patient should be admitted and administered intravenous antibiotics aimed at a staphylococcus aureus infection. Hand therapy is started immediately. In case of a fulminant infection with a necrotic flexor tendon and sheath, the finger must be opened according to Bruner. After necrosectomy and rinsing of the wound, the skin is closed with as little as possible sutures.

SEPTIC ARTHRITIS

GENERAL

An infected joint usually becomes stiff, with any movement being painful. The soft tissue around the joint is red and swollen. Joint narrowing, cartilage erosion and osteolysis can only be seen on X-ray imaging weeks later.

The cause can be a bacterial infection through a small wound or a thorn, or due to bacteremia of an infection elsewhere in the body. Non-bacterial joint inflammation is possible, whereby gout, pseudo-gout and rheumatic disease are seen most often.

TREATMENT BY HAND SURGEON

Opening of the joint with thorough rinsing, after which the joint is immobilized and the patient treated with intravenous antibiotics.

PALM INFECTIONS, PHLEGMON

GENERAL

This is usually caused by penetrating wounds or injections, or sometimes only small wounds in diabetic patients. A tendon sheath infection can extend to the palm lodges (Figure 14.1).

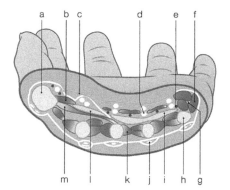

a.	os metacarpal of the thumb
b.	thenar muscles
c.	aponeurosis palmaris
d.	flexor tendons
e.	neurovascular bundle
f.	hypothenar muscles
g.	hypothenar space
h.	fifth metacarpal
i.	mid palmar space
j.	extensor tendons
k.	interosseous muscles
l.	thenar space
m.	m. adductor pollicis

Figure 14.1 Cross section palm. a: os metacarpal of the thumb, b: thenar muscles, c: aponeurosis palmaris, d: flexor tendons, e: neurovascular bundle, f: hypothenar muscles, g: hypothenar space, h: fifth metacarpal, i: mid palmar space, j: extensor tendons, k: interosseous muscles, l: thenar space, m: m. adductor pollicis.

TREATMENT

Exploration and drainage must be carried out as a matter of urgency. The patient should receive intravenous antibiotics. There are four potential localizations of an abscess:

1. **The interdigital space**. This will cause the fingers to be abducted due to swelling.
2. **Midpalmar space**. The concavity of the palm has disappeared and the mobility of the middle and ring fingers are painful and limited. The infection can quickly spread to the forearm to the space of Parona, located between the mm. FDP and the m. pronator quadratus.
3. **Thenar space**. Causes a swelling over the thenar region and the first interdigital space.
4. **Hypothenar space**. This is rare. There will be a swelling of the hypothenar.

VIRAL INFECTIONS: HERPES, ORF

- Herpes is caused by the herpes simplex virus. Vesicles arise two to 14 days after contact. The infection is self-limiting and surgical intervention is contraindicated. Acyclovir can accelerate healing and prevent recurrence.
- Orf is a viral infection caused by close contact with an infected sheep or goat. After three to seven days, a solid, painless tumor appears. The disease itself is self-limiting and here too surgical intervention is contraindicated.

For both, short-term immobilization and elevation is useful.

Combustion and high pressure spray injury

THERMAL COMBUSTION AND FREEZING

POINTS OF ATTENTION

There is a chance of physical abuse when it involves children. Consider a consultation by the pediatrician. It is best not to use Flammazine or Flammacerium when the depth of the wound is yet to be determined. Instead, cover the wound with paraffin tulle.

PATIENT HISTORY

A burn is a partial or full thickness damage to the skin, caused by the action of heat, electricity or a chemical reaction. Be aware of an inhalation trauma and consider bronchoscopy if there is reason to do so. The severity of the burn depends on size, depth and localization. The size is expressed in the percentage of total body surface area (TBSA). The palm of the hand is considered 1% TBSA. The depth of the burn depends on the temperature of the source, the nature of the material and the duration of the burn. The thickness of the skin is of influence: a dorsal hand burn is usually deeper than a volar burn. Ask about the duration of cooling.

PHYSICAL EXAMINATION

Estimate the depth and extent of the burn. In partial thickness burns, there is a distinction between a superficial and deep dermal burn. In the case of superficial burn the skin is red, sometimes with blisters, there is a rapid capillary refill and the patient is in a lot of pain. This burn heals spontaneously within two weeks. A deep dermal injury shows a cloudy aspect of the skin, sometimes with blisters. The pain and capillary refill are moderate. This burn does not heal within two weeks and can lead to severe scars and contraction. Full thickness burns can have a white/yellow, reddish brown to black skin colour. The skin can be parchment-like. There is no sensibility and no capillary refill. Spontaneous healing is possible, but this can take months and is accompanied by disabling contractures.

TREATMENT

Small burns can be treated conservatively with paraffin tulle gras. Larger burns should be covered with Flammazine or Flammacerium. Significant burns deserve the attention of a hand surgeon. An escharotomy should be considered in case of circular burns. If the burn to the hand is part of a large burn, then referral to a burns center is indicated.

CHEMICAL BURNS

POINTS OF ATTENTION

Chemical injuries can be caused by solids, liquids and vapors or gases. The severity depends on the concentration, acidity, penetrating properties and duration of exposure to the agent. Alkaline substances appear innocent at first, but can create full thickness burns (i.e. cement). Some substances give an eczema-like reaction that is difficult to distinguish from a burn. Treatment should be given in consultation with your National Poison Control Center.

PATIENT HISTORY

The following is important:

- the exact nature of the chemical
- the duration of exposure
- has the burn been rinsed and for how long
- the use of a specific antidote

Alkaline substances often cause more damage than acids, except for hydrogen fluoride (HF; used for etching glass and high pressure cleaning of walls). The latter leads to very painful, deep necrosis until neutralized with calcium gluconate and can be fatal in high tissue concentrations.

PHYSICAL EXAMINATION

As always, estimate the depth and size of the burn. Hydrogen fluoride affects the nail bed.

ADDITIONAL EXAMINATION

In the case of a severe hydrogen fluoride injury, serum calcium levels should be obtained.

TREATMENT

Rinse with large volumes of water as soon as possible (< ten minutes). For alkaline substances, rinse for a long time (at least one hour). Consult a hand surgeon. In the case of hydrogen fluoride injection, treat with calcium gluconate burn gel (10% with DMSO) and subcutaneous injection with a 10% solution of calcium gluconate (multiple injections of 0.1–0.2 mL into the wound). Give a Biers block with calcium gluconate solution. In case of phosphorus burns, irrigate with 1% copper sulfate solution. In case of tar burns leave tar in place or remove with toluene. Think of systemic effects that can be caused by the agent (to the liver, kidneys, heart). In the case of significant burns, refer to a burns center.

ELECTRICITY BURNS

POINTS OF ATTENTION

Electricity burns are always deep. There may be an additional thermal burn due to the heat of burnt clothing. If a fasciotomy of endangered muscle compartments is performed, the sudden release of myoglobin from the damaged skeletal muscle can cause renal insufficiency. Cardiac complications can occur in case of high-voltage injuries and lightning strikes.

PATIENT HISTORY

Ask about the height of the voltage (low voltage or high voltage), the frequency and the duration of exposure (domestic power supply carry 220 Volt, 50 Hz, industrial power >1000 Volt).

PHYSICAL EXAMINATION

Look at the entry and exit point (sometimes in one hand, out the other). High voltage injury (>1000 Volt) can cause a massive coagulation and cause necrosis with circulation problems of an extremity (compartment syndrome). Investigate the circulation of the distal extremity.

ADDITIONAL EXAMINATION

Patients should have 24-hour ECG monitoring in the event of high voltage burns. Additionally, blood chemistry and coagulation should be examined, including CPK and LDH.

TREATMENT

Small lesions (size of millimeters) can be treated conservatively with tulle, Flammazine or Flammacerium. Larger areas limited to the hand: consult a hand surgeon for escharotomy, fasciotomy and secondary closure of the defects.

HIGH PRESSURE WASHER INJURY

POINTS OF ATTENTION

The wound may be very small or invisible. Do not use Oberst anesthesia or pressure bandages.

PATIENT HISTORY

These are rare but very serious injuries. Often the index finger of the non-dominant hand is applied during cleaning of the nozzle head or covering a hole in the hose. Under high pressure, foreign material (oil, grease, paint, solvents) is injected into the finger.

The material may end up deep inside the finger (flexor tendon sheath) and migrate proximally due to local pressure (into the palm/wrist). Chemical reaction and secondary infection can lead to necrosis of the whole finger or hand.

Physical examination

Often a small entry wound in the pulp. Initially patients show few symptoms. At a later stage there is evident swelling, pain and stiffness.

Imaging

An X-ray of the area injected, only if the material is radiopaque.

Treatment

The patient should be quickly referred to a hand surgeon for decompression and removal of the material. Elevate the hand.

Complex regional pain syndrome type I

C.H. EMMELOT
rehabilitation specialist

GENERAL

Complex regional pain syndrome type I (CRPS I) is, according to the most recent taxonomy, a disorder of unknown origin which can manifest itself as an acute problem. It does not constitute a specific disease but is rather a number of symptoms that occur frequently in the same combinations. One distinguishes a hot and cold phase whose symptomatology, however, can also be mixed.

POINTS OF ATTENTION

CRPS I will only be considered if other causes for a autonomic dysfunction are excluded. Look for neurological malfunction. A simple CTS can cause vegetative disturbances (CRPS type II, a dysregulation based on nerve damage).

PATIENT HISTORY

Is there a (trivial) trauma? Cold intolerance is a sensitive symptom. The pain experienced in CRPS is described as a burning sensation. Although only 50% of the CRPS patients experience increased sweat secretion, it is suggestive for CRPS.

Additionally, patients experience allodynia: sensory stimulation that normally does not cause pain is now experienced as painful and can give violent reactions.

DOI: 10.1201/9781003313540-16

PHYSICAL EXAMINATION

The diagnosis is based on clinical symptoms. An acute CRPS is characterized by major symptoms: swelling, stiffness, pain, functio laesa and rubor. Autonomic dysregulation can express itself as increased sweating, discoloration, abnormal temperature and trophic disorders such as abnormal growth of hairs and nails.

DIFFERENTIAL DIAGNOSIS

The acute 'warm CRPS' should be distinguished from:

- acute inflammatory processes
- (poly)neuropathy (as in diabetes mellitus and carpal tunnel syndrome)
- venous thrombosis, thrombophlebitis
- local contusion with hematoma formation
- compartment syndrome
- intra-arterial administration of hard drugs

The 'cold CRPS' should be distinguished from other types of vegetative dysregulations as seen in:

- arterial insufficiency and embolism, Raynaud's disease
- post-traumatic vasospasm
- glomus tumor
- osteoid osteoma

ADDITIONAL EXAMINATION

For the diagnosis of CRPS, no additional examination is indicated. The diagnosis is made on clinical grounds and after exclusion of other, more specific and treatment-eligible conditions. The following can be requested to rule out other conditions:

X-ray: fractures, foreign body, bone tumor (e.g. osteoid osteoma).
Laboratory examination: inflammatory parameters for differentiation of abscess, gangrene, phlegmon, erysipelas and arthritis.
Ultrasound: detection of fluid collection (bursitis, synovitis, deep vein thrombosis, etc.)
Neurophysiological examination: to exclude neuropathy or nerve compression.

Index

Page numbers in *italics* indicate figures.

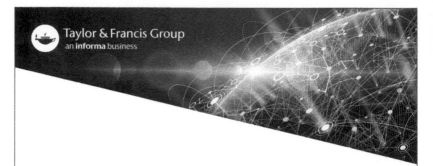

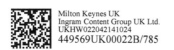